Healing Salves

25 Homemade Recipes for Health and Healing

Table of Contents

Introduction

I wish to thank and congratulate you on downloading *"Healing Salve: 25 Homemade Herbal Salve Recipes for Health and Healing."* You will find that this collection of healthy herbal salve recipes are very easy to follow and prepare. These are simple recipes that only have a few ingredients per recipe, so you will not have to go into any great expense at all to get the ingredients you need to make these salves.

Just keep in mind that I am not saying that you should self-diagnose yourself on any health issue you may have. You need to first go and seek professional advice from your doctor about any kind of medical condition you are suffering from.

You will find that these salve recipes will work wonders on basic skin irritations, and will have your skin looking healthy in no time. You will feel good in knowing you are using a product that is natural and has no additives in it or man-made chemicals. I hope that you and your loved ones will enjoy using this collection of homemade herbal healing salves for many years to come!

Chapter 1.   Basic Herbal Healing Salve

To introduce you into the world of healing herbal salves we will start off with a very simple recipe for a healing salve.

1. *Healing Salve*

Ingredients:

- sixteen ounces of base oil such as almond oil, coconut oil or olive oil

- one and a half ounces of beeswax

- essential oils chosen by you for their particular healing properties

When you are making homemade herbal salves they usually include fat carrier oil and herbal oils. The essential oils you choose will be added after the process of heating the base oil, or infused oil with beeswax. After this has been removed from heat then the essential oils are added.

Supplies you will need to make your herbal salves are:

- herb infused oil with desired herbs of your choice

- beeswax

- jars or tins to store your salve in

- cheesecloth to drain out oil and separate herbs from oil

- essential oils that you choose to you in your salve

Choosing Herbs for Your Salve:

To begin the first thing that you must decide is what particular herbs you want to use to make your infused herbal oil. Take precaution when handling the ingredients. Do not overwhelm yourself when you are trying to decide what herbs you want to include in your infused oil. You would be best to start with 3-5 herbs. It is a very good idea to do the research and make sure that they are compatible with any medications that you are taking.

Making Your Herbal Infused Oil: Once you have chosen the herbs that you are going to use to make your herbal infused oil the next thing you must do in the process is to choose what kind of carrier oil you are going to use. I myself prefer to use coconut oil for my salves because it has great properties and is nice and firm. Sometimes I will mix it with a bit of olive oil as this is great for the skin.

When you have decided how much product you are making this will help you to decide on the size of containers you will need in order to store it in. I like to use small canning jars as they are perfect for when you have to put them into a double broiler to heat them. Fill your canning jars half-full of herbs. I will add more of my key herb than the rest of them.

Now add in your choice of carrier oil to heat-proof bowl along with the herbs. Heat over low heat in a double broiler with water half-way up the outside of the bowl that contains the oil and herbs. Heat oil for about three hours then allow to cool and stress oil through cheesecloth into another collection container. Discard the herbs. Add the oil back into the heat-proof bowl with beeswax and heat until the wax has melted. Add into your choice of storage containers that have secure lids.

Chapter 2. Tips, Suggestions and Salve Recipes

If you would like your salve to have a thick consistency then all you need to do is just add more beeswax to make it thicker. Beeswax is not the only wax available but I do find that it is fairly priced and works well in making salves.

All you have to do is add a little beeswax into your infused oil to make a nice salve paste. A great way for you to use herbal products is to add them to your salves. Of course it is not a must that you use herbs in your salves the choice of course is up to yourself.

You will find that there is room for you to create your own special salves using different combinations of ingredients to suit your personal needs and taste. When you change the amount of an ingredient in your salve you will change the outcome at the end. So do not fear trying adding or reducing new ingredients to make your own special salve. Don't be afraid to use the recipes for salves below as a base for making your own special salves.

1. *Orange & Wintergreen Creamy Body Salve*

Ingredients:

- one cup of coconut butter
- half a cup of coconut oil
- half a cup of Jojoba oil
- twelve drops of orange essential oil
- twelve drops of wintergreen essential oil

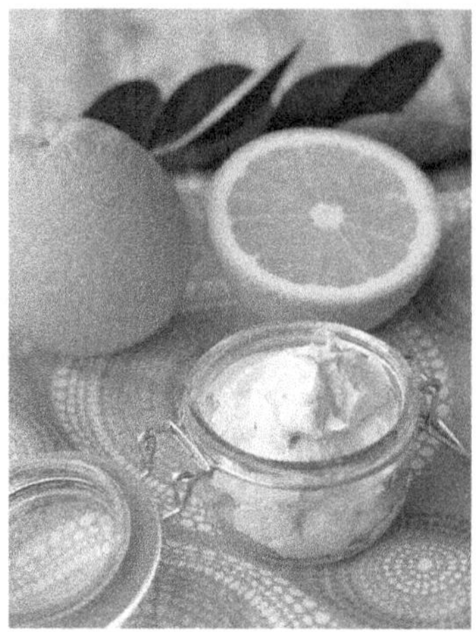

Directions:

Melt the coconut butter along with coconut oil and Jojoba oil, in a double broiler over medium heat. Once it is melted remove from heat and add in your essential oils and blend well.

Place mix into the fridge until it is almost hard, remove and whip with hand mixer until fluffy. Place in container for storage and put back into fridge for another ten minutes. Remove from fridge and secure on the lid. Store this salve for up to ten months. It will work great on sore aching muscles and dry skin.

2. Basic Calendula Salve

Ingredients:

- two and a half ounces of Calendula, dried

- six ounces of almond oil

- one quarter of a cup of beeswax

Directions:

Add all of your ingredients into a double broiler heating over simmer for three hours. Remove from heat and stress the oil using a cheesecloth. Discard the herbs and collect oil in container.

Add your collected herbal infused oil and put into heat-proof bowl along with beeswax and reheat in broiler over medium heat until the beeswax is melted. Allow to cool enough so then you can put into storage containers. Seal with secure lid. Store this salve in a cool dark place for up to a year.

3. *Lavender & Coconut Muscle Salve*

Ingredients:

- half a cup of coconut oil
- three tablespoons of Shea butter
- one quarter of a cup of beeswax
- half a teaspoon of vitamin E oil
- 20 drops of lavender essential oil

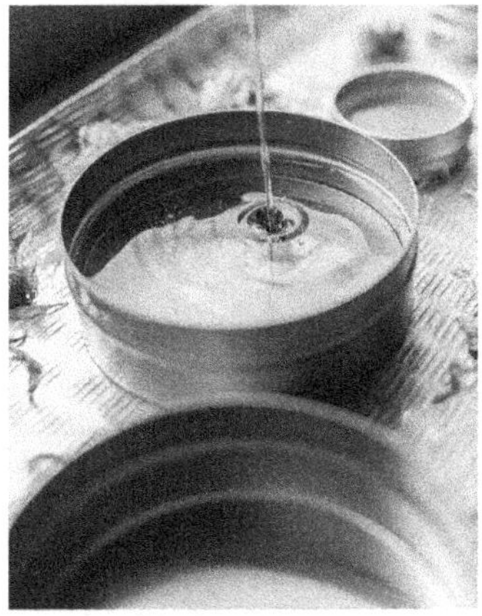

Directions:

In a double broiler over medium heat add in coconut oil, Shea butter and beeswax. Stir until it is melted then remove from heat. Add in the vitamin E oil and essential oil and mix well. Add to chosen storage containers and secure lid. You can store this salve up to six months.

4. Spearmint Pain Reliever Salve

Ingredients:

- half a cup of coconut oil

- two ounces of beeswax

- 15 drops of cinnamon essential oil

- 20 drops of camphor essential oil

- 20 drops of spearmint essential oil

- eight drops of clove essential oil

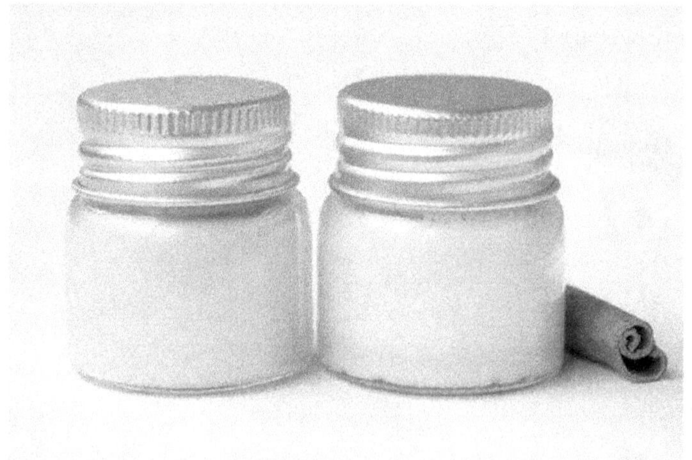

Directions:

Add to your double broiler the coconut oil, and beeswax over medium heat, stir until mix is melted. Remove from the heat and add in your essential oils and blend mix well. Add to tins or jars and seal lid. Allow to cool before you use it. This is a great salve that will help relieve pain in sore muscles and even headaches.

5. *Arnica Pain Relieving Salve*

Ingredients:

- one cup of coconut oil
- one ounce of Arnica, dried
- one quarter of a teaspoon of vitamin E
- 20 drops of Marjoram essential oil
- one quarter of a cup of beeswax

Directions:

In a double broiler add your coconut oil, along with the Arnica and simmer for two hours. Remove from heat and stress the oil using a cheesecloth. Collect oil in container and discard the herbs.

Add oil along with beeswax back into broiler over medium heat, stir until melted. Remove from heat and add in your essential oil and vitamin E and mix well. Add mix to containers and seal lid. Keep in a dark cool place, this salve will last for up to a year. It works well for aching muscles and bones.

6. Basic Comfrey Salve

Ingredients:

- two and a half ounces of comfrey leaves, dried

- one cup of almond oil

- one quarter of a cup of beeswax

- twelve drops of Camphor essential oil

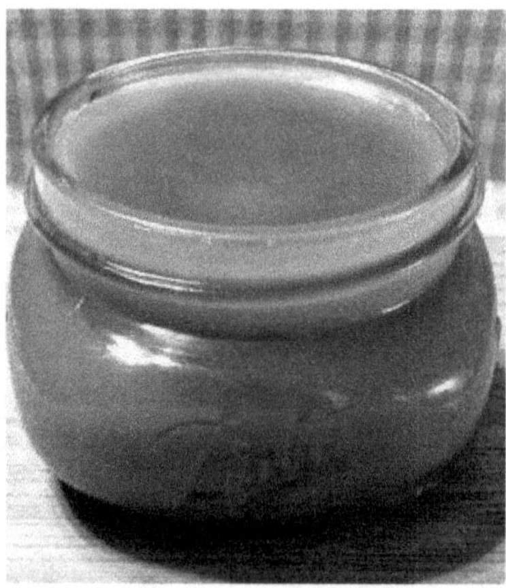

Directions:

Place the comfrey leaves and almond oil into double broiler over simmer for an hour. Remove from heat and stress the oil through cheesecloth. Collect oil and discard the herbs. Add oil back into the double broiler with beeswax over medium heat, stir until melted.

Remove from heat add in the essential oil and mix well. Add mix to containers and seal with secure lid. This is a great salve to help with skin wounds, or skin problems. First clean wound with hydrogen peroxide then apply the salve.

7. Cracked Foot Heel Salve

Ingredients:

- one quarter of a cup of coconut oil

- one quarter of a cup of Shea butter

- one quarter of a cup of Magnesium flakes with two tablespoons of boiling water

- twelve drops of oregano essential oil

- fifteen drops of peppermint essential oil

Directions:

In a small bowl add two tablespoons of boiling water and add in the Magnesium flakes and mix. Allow to cool. In a double broiler add in the Shea butter, beeswax, and coconut oil, stir until melted over medium heat. Remove from heat and add into a bowl and blend well. Add in the Magnesium paste.

After it as been well-blended put into the fridge for twenty minutes. Remove from fridge and re-blend mix. Store mix for up to eight weeks in the fridge. Use this salve on dry or cracked feet at night. For the best results you should first exfoliate the skin from your feet before you apply the salve. Repeat this process until your feet are cleared up.

8. *Calendula & Comfrey Salve*

Ingredients:

- half an ounce of Calendula, dried

- half an ounce of Comfrey, dried

- one cup of cold pressed olive oil

- half an ounce of beeswax

- five vitamin E capsules

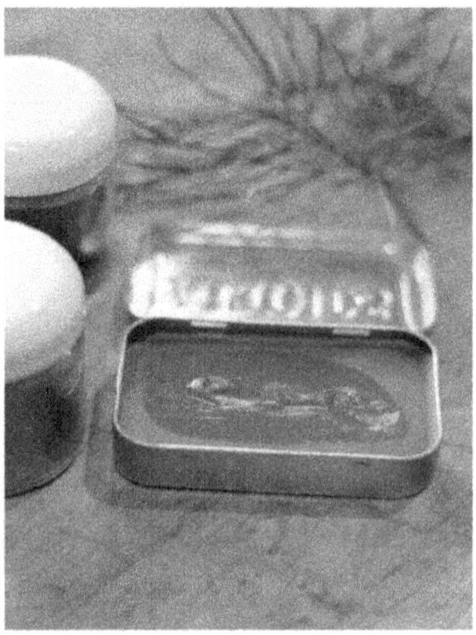

Directions:

In your double broiler add in oil and herbs cook on low for 30 minutes, stirring occasionally. Allow the mix to cool then stress it through cheesecloth collect oil and discard the herbs. Add collected oil back into the double broiler with beeswax and over medium heat stir until melted. Remove from heat and add in vitamin E capsules. Add to jars and seal with secure lid.

9. *Polk Root & Blood Root Salve to Help in Treating Skin Cancer*

Ingredients:

- one tablespoon of Polk root

- one tablespoon of Blood-Root

- one tablespoon of activated charcoal powder

- one tablespoon of Pascalite clay

- one tablespoon of almond oil

- one tablespoon of zinc chloride, crystal or liquid

- one teaspoon of wood tar

Directions:

Add two tablespoons of warm water if you are using the crystal form of zinc chloride and mix until dissolved then set aside. Mix blood-root and Polk-root with almond oil and charcoal powder. Add in the zinc and mix well. Heat mix in a double broiler for 30 minutes on low heat. Add in the Pascalite clay and wood tar, mix well into a paste.

If it seems too thick just add in a couple of more drops of almond oil. Apply this salve to the area of skin that has cancer lesions and cover with a gauze for 12 hours. After the treatment wash the area with soap and water then clean with hydrogen peroxide. Apply this treatment every 2-3 days. The cancer lesions may disappear after one to five months. You may experience stinging or burning this is normal.

10. *Blood-Root Black Salve for Skin Cancer*

Ingredients:

- half a cup of blood-root, powdered

- half a cup of white flour

- half a cup of zinc chloride, crystals or liquid

- two cups of hot water

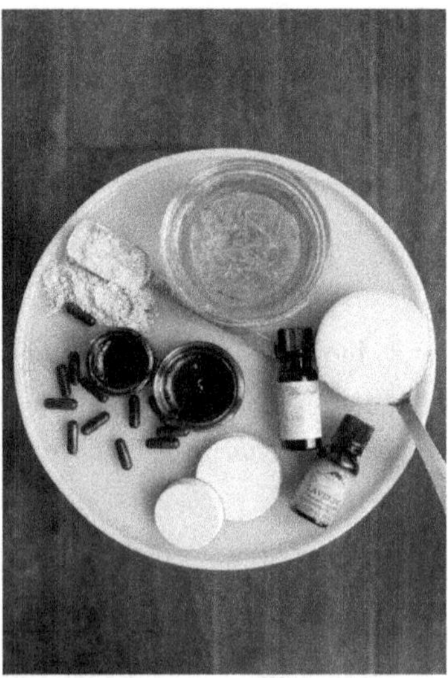

Directions:

Add all of your ingredients and mix except for water. Add to double broiler mix and water and mix well. This is a treatment used for skin cancer lesions. This is a good treatment for the skin cancer lesions that are at the top of the skin or exposed.

Once the mix has cooled then apply to area on skin where the cancer is. Do not try to pull off lesions they will fall out in 10 days time. You can add Vaseline around the outer rim of where you applied the salve so the mix does not irritate your surrounding skin.

11. Healing Echinacea Root Salve

Ingredients:

- one cup of almond oil
- one teaspoon of plantain leaf
- one teaspoon of echinacea root
- one quarter of a cup of beeswax
- one teaspoon of Calendula flowers
- one teaspoon of comfrey leaf
- one teaspoon of rosemary leaf
- one tablespoon of grapefruit seed extract
- one teaspoon of yarrow flowers
- twelve drops of peppermint essential oil

Directions:

In a double broiler add in almond oil and herbs in a heat-proof bowl, water should be in broiler halfway up the outside of the bowl. Heat your oil and herbs over low heat for three hours. Allow to cool so that you are able to stress the oil with cheesecloth, collect oil in a container then discard the herbs.

 Add the oil back into heat-proof bowl along with beeswax, reheat over medium heat until the beeswax is melted. Remove from heat and add in your essential oils and mix well. Pour into small containers this salve works well on dry and chapped lips.

12. *Pregnancy Stretch-Mark Salve*

Ingredients:

- one quarter of a cup of almond oil

- one quarter of a cup of Shea butter

- five tablespoons of Apricot Kernel oil

- one tablespoon of Calendula flowers

- one quarter of a teaspoon of ginger-root, dried

Directions:

Add almond oil along with dry ginger-root, and Calendula flowers to double broiler in a heat-proof bowl. Simmer and mix for about three hours then remove from heat. Stress the oil in cheesecloth, collect oil in another container, discard the herbs.

Add the oil back into the heat-proof bowl add in the Shea butter and heat until the Shea butter is melted and mix well. Add mix to glass jar, this can be used during pregnancy and after.

13. Black-Drawing Salve

Ingredients:

- four tablespoons of comfrey

- three teaspoons of Shea butter

- three tablespoons of coconut oil

- one tablespoon of honey

- three tablespoons of Kaolin clay

- three tablespoons of Calendula, dried

- two tablespoons of charcoal powder, activated

- twenty drops of lavender essential oil

- two capsules of vitamin E

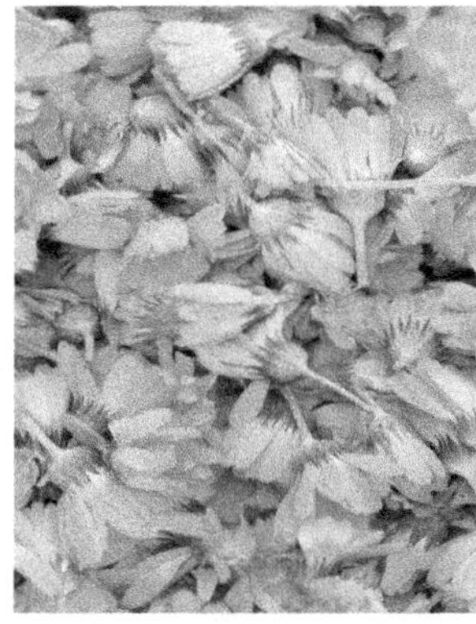

Directions:

Mix Calendula, comfrey and oil. Add to a jar and leave for five days. Each day shake the jar a few times a day. Then strain through a cheesecloth, discarding the herbs, and adding the infused oil to double broiler.

Add in also beeswax, Shea butter and vitamin E over medium heat until it is melted and mix well. Remove from heat and add in essential oil, charcoal powder, and kaolin clay and mix well. Store in glass jars that have secure lids. This salve works great on cuts and splinters.

14. Dandelion Salve Recipe

Ingredients:

- one bowl of dried dandelions
- one cup of grapeseed oil
- twelve drops of lavender essential oil
- one quarter of a cup of beeswax

Directions:

In a double broiler boil the dandelions and oil over simmer. Heat for about three hours on simmer. Then use a cheesecloth to stress the oil and collect it in container, discard the dandelions.

Put the oil back into the heat-proof bowl in double broiler and add in beeswax, heat over medium heat until the beeswax has melted, remove from heat and stir. Add in your essential oil and mix well. Store in a glass jar with secure lid and keep in the fridge up to two months.

15. Capsaicin Pain Relief Salve

Ingredients:

- one cup of grapeseed oil

- one quarter of a cup of beeswax

- three tablespoons of cayenne powder

Directions:

Add cayenne pepper, grapeseed oil, to a double broiler over medium heat then add in beeswax. Heat over medium heat until the beeswax is melted. Remove from heat and then put in the fridge and chill for ten minutes. Remove from fridge and whisk then add to glass jar with secure lid. This should keep for two months if you keep in the fridge.

16. Extra-Strength Pain Relief Salve

Ingredients:

- one quarter of a cup of beeswax

- three cups of grapeseed oil

- four tablespoons of Habanero powder

Directions:

Add in Habanero powder to a double broiler along with grapeseed oil over medium heat then add in the beeswax and stir leave on until the beeswax is melted. Remove from heat and put in the fridge for ten minutes. Remove and whisk then put in glass jar and seal with lid and place back in your fridge for up to two months.

17. Cinnamon & Turmeric Pain Reducer Salve

Ingredients:

- three cups of grapeseed oil

- four tablespoons of turmeric

- one quarter of a cup of beeswax

- four tablespoons of cinnamon, ground

- four tablespoons of cayenne, ground

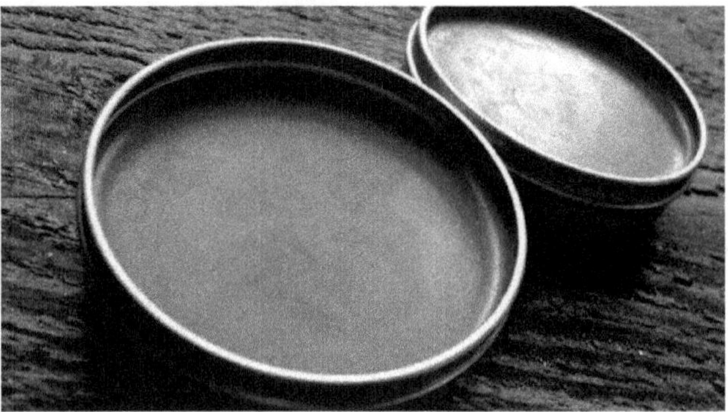

Directions:

Mix in a bowl cinnamon, turmeric, and cayenne. In a double broiler add in grapeseed oil and cinnamon mix and stir until well-blended. Heat over medium heat then add in beeswax and stir and cook until the beeswax is melted then remove from heat.

Put in the fridge to chill for ten minutes. Remove from fridge and whisk. Add to glass jar and place back into the fridge. This is a great salve that will help improve your circulation, and will help get the vitamins your bones need as they will deliver oxygen to your bones. This is good to use especially if you suffer from osteoarthritis.

18. *Salve for Aching & Sore Muscles*

Ingredients:

- two tablespoons of beeswax

- one quarter of a cup of almond oil

- one quarter of a cup of coconut oil

- one quarter of a teaspoon of cinnamon, ground

- one quarter of a teaspoon of black pepper, freshly ground

- 25 drops of peppermint essential oil

- 20 drops of eucalyptus essential oil

- 20 drops of clove oil

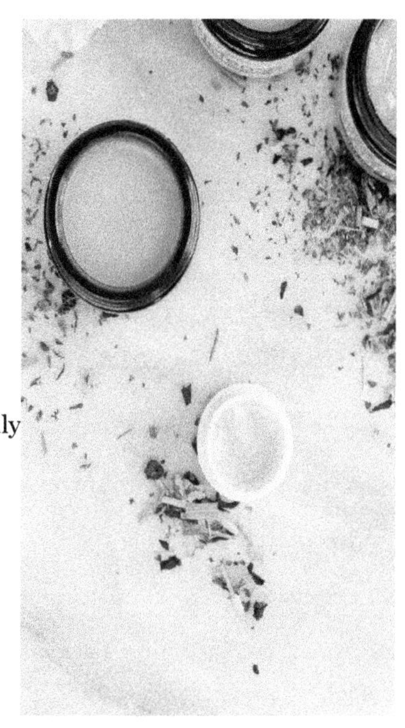

Directions:

In a double broiler in a heat-proof bowl add your base oils—almond oil and coconut oil. Add in cinnamon and black pepper. Bring water to a boil then reduce to simmer. Remove from heat after 20 minutes and allow to steep.

Allow to steep for an hour and then re-heat adding beeswax over medium heat. Heat and stir until the beeswax has melted. Remove from heat then add in the essential oils and mix well. Let sit at room temperature for three hours then apply this salve onto your sore muscles directly.

19. *Herbal Salve*

Ingredients:

- one quarter cup of almond oil

- one quarter cup of coconut oil

- one quarter cup of beeswax

- eight drops of grapefruit essential oil

- ten drops of rose essential oil

- ten drops of peppermint essential oil

Directions:

In a small pot heat your base oils and beeswax over medium heat until the beeswax has melted. Remove from heat and add in the essential oils and mix well. Then add to glass jar with secure lid.

20. *Raw Honey & Aloe Vera Burn Salve*

Ingredients:

- three tablespoons of coconut oil

- one quarter of a cup of raw honey

- three tablespoons of aloe vera

Directions:

Mix your ingredients in a small pot over medium heat, use a wooden spoon to mix. Remove from heat and add to glass jar. Clean the area of burned skin first using some apple cider vinegar. Using this treatment can help to recover vitamins to the burned skin and will help restore the pH balance of your skin. After you have applied the salve cover it with gauze. Do not use this treatment on serious burns—seek medical attention.

21. *Lavender & Chamomile Hand Salve*

Ingredients:

- one quarter of a cup of beeswax

- one quarter of a cup of almond oil

- one quarter of a cup of coconut oil

- one quarter of a cup of lavender, dried

- one quarter of a cup of chamomile, dried

- ten drops of lavender essential oil

- five drops of Eucalyptus essential oil

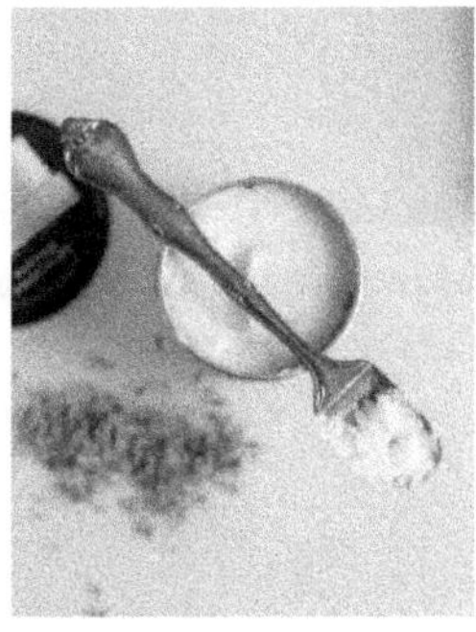

Directions:

In a saucepan over medium heat add in your almond oil, coconut oil, lavender, and chamomile. Stir until it becomes hot. Lower heat to simmer and continue to cook for another hour.

Remove from heat then stress the oil through a cheesecloth and discard the herbs. Add the oil back into saucepan along with beeswax over medium heat until the beeswax has melted. Remove from heat and add in essential oils, mix well. Add to glass jar first allow it to cool for a bit. Seal jar with a secure lid.

22. *Chickweed Oil & Comfrey Salve*

Ingredients:

- half a cup of chickweed oil

- two ounces of comfrey, dried leaves

- twenty drops of lavender essential oil

- one quarter cup of beeswax

Directions:

In a double broiler add the chickweed oil and the comfrey leaves bring to a boil. Reduce to simmer and continue to cook for another hour. Remove from heat and then stress the oil through cheesecloth, discard herbs.

Add the oil back into double broiler along with beeswax over medium heat. Heat until the beeswax is melted, then remove from heat add in the essential oil and mix well. Add to glass jar with secure lid and keep in the fridge.

23. *Healing Salve*

Ingredients:

- one cup of coconut oil

- one cup of almond oil

- two ounces of comfrey leaf, dried

- three tablespoons of plantain leaf, dried

- one teaspoon of echinacea root

- one quarter of a cup of beeswax

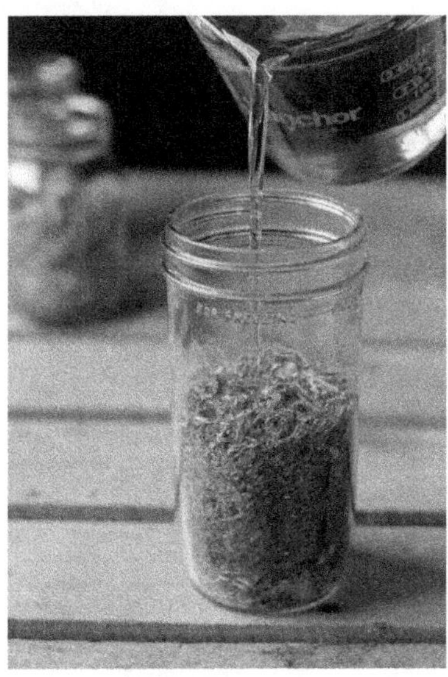

Directions:

Add your herbs to your base oils in a double broiler and bring to a boil then reduce to a simmer for one hour. Remove from heat then stress the oil through cheesecloth.

Discard the herbs and put the oil back into the double broiler along with the beeswax over medium heat. Heat until the beeswax has melted and remove from heat. Add in the echinacea root and mix well. Add to small tins for storing. Use this salve on poison ivy, diaper rash, or other injuries of the skin.

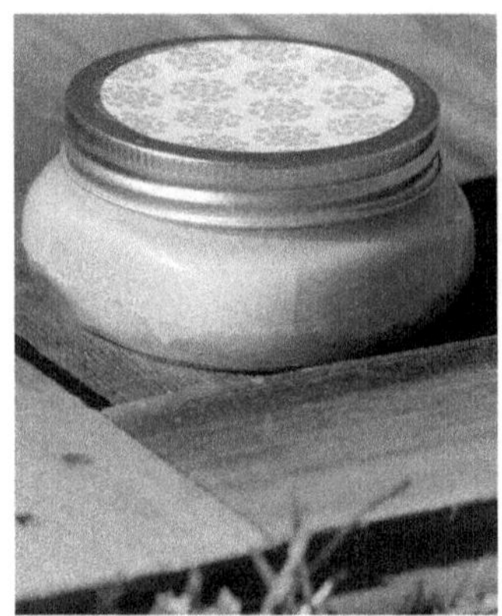

24. Vapor Rub

Ingredients:

- half a cup of almond oil

- one quarter of a cup of beeswax

- twelve drops of cinnamon essential oil

- twelve drops of rosemary essential oil

- twenty drops of eucalyptus essential oil

- twenty drops of peppermint essential oil

Directions:

In a double broiler add in the almond oil and the beeswax over medium heat. Heat until the wax has melted and stir. Remove from heat and add in the essential oils and mix well. Put into small storing tins. This can be used on chest to help ease congestion and coughing.

25. *Comfort & Soothing Salve*

Ingredients:

- half a cup of grapeseed oil

- half a cup of coconut oil

- half a tablespoon of vitamin E oil

- one quarter of a cup of beeswax

- eight drops of Rose, Melaleuca, Cypress, Frankincense and Eucalyptus essential oils

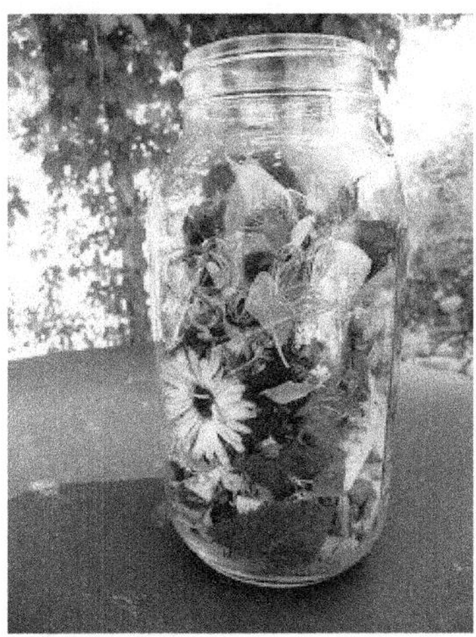

Directions:

In a double broiler add in the base oils—grapeseed and coconut along with the beeswax over medium heat. Cook until the beeswax is melted stirring occasionally. Remove from heat and add in the vitamin E oil and essential oils, mix well. Add to jars and allow to set for a couple of hours before use. Apply this salve to skin or chest area.

Conclusion

I hope my collection of salves will bring great comfort and healing to you and your loved ones. This is a great way to spend time with a loved ones when preparing these wonderful salves. Get comfort from knowing that these products are natural and are not filled with all kinds of additives and chemicals.

These are wonderful organic healing aids that you and your family will grow to love using. Not only will you enjoy the healing benefits of these salves but you are going to save yourself a great deal of money when you are no longer spending a small fortune on man-made chemical filled products.

I want to thank you again for downloading my book it means a great deal to me that you are supporting my work. I would be so delighted to read a review by you of my book on Amazon. Take care and happy healing salve making!